HEALTHY LIVING VIA RAW FOODS:

Returning to raw foods diet for a healthy eating experience

By

Jose M. Butts

Table of Contents

INTRODUCTION

Humans had been consuming fresh fruit, veggies, and nuts for 10-50,000 years or more before we developed fire, tools, and equipment to slaughter animals.

Eating fresh fruits and veggies isn't the latest trendy diet or the new South Beach Diet. Believe it or not, people have been eating this way long before they were consuming packaged junky meals. We didn't have access to most sorts of meals. We were scavengers, gathering fruits and eating veggies was a delicacy. Nuts were also consumed for protein. It was either that or starving.

Humans ate these fruits as it is, with no additives, and no preparation. One and a half million years ago humanity discovered how to cook. So for a half million years, we ate the food uncooked, as it was meant. We are the only creatures on the earth that boil their food. Eating meat quadrupled the caloric intake of man, which made it simpler to hunt and have the energy to perform what has to be done.

Today, we have access to any sort of food we desire at our fingertips. We may get Oolong tea (which must be chosen on cliffs in china) via the internet. You would assume that because we have progressed this far, we would be superhuman, so healthy we would be living 500 years. Not so sadly.
In fact, in some areas, we have poorer health presently. Some of us are acquiring malignancies at an early age. Some of us are dying of heart disease or weight. We are not eating appropriately. We are cramming our faces with hydrogenated oils, false goods, excessive salt, and sugary meals. It is horrible. We are gaining weight at an alarming pace and looking awful. It shows in the skin, sags of fat, lethargic attitude, gloomy appearance, lack of sexual desire, etc. I wonder how long we would live if we adopted the diet of the Japanese.

What individuals need to know is that eating fat-free or sugar-free meals isn't going to help. It isn't going to help if you load your face with snack wells instead of Oreos. What will help is to radically modify what you consume. Remember, you are what you eat, therefore eat the correct stuff and embrace a raw foods diet and it will show in your body, mind, and soul.

What is the Raw Food Diet?

Have you started hearing about the Raw Food Diet? It's gaining popularity and buzz, not just as a diet to lose weight, but as a diet for a long and healthy life. We eat so much processed food that we don't even stop to think about what we're putting into our bodies, and how far we've come nutritionally from our ancestral, agrarian roots.

A raw food diet means consuming food in its natural, unprocessed form. There are several common-sense rationales for why this is a good idea. Processing and cooking food can take so much of the basic nutritional value away. Think of some of the conventional wisdom you've heard about for years, such as: If you cook pasta just to the al dente (or medium) stage, it will have more calories, yes, but it will have more nutritional value in it than if you cooked it to a well-done stage. Or you probably remember hearing not to peel carrots or potatoes too deeply, because most of the nutrients and values are just under the surface.

The raw food diet means eating unprocessed, uncooked, organic, whole foods, such as fruits, vegetables, nuts, seeds, legumes, dried fruits, seaweed, etc. It means a diet that is at least 75% uncooked! Cooking takes out flavor and nutrition from vegetables and fruits.

A raw food diet means eating more the way our ancient ancestors did. Our healthier, more fit ancestors. They cooked very little and certainly didn't cook or process fruits and vegetables. They ate them RAW. Their water wasn't from a tap; it was natural, spring water. Maybe they drank some coconut milk on occasion.

Doesn't it just make sense that this is how our bodies were meant to eat? It's a way of eating that's in harmony with the planet and harmony with our metabolism. Our bodies are meant to work and need to work to be efficient. That means exercise, certainly, but it also means eating natural, raw foods that require less energy to digest them.

The cooking process (i.e., heating meals over 116°F) is considered to deactivate food enzymes.
People who adopt the raw diet utilize specialized procedures to prepare meals. Which include sprouting seeds, grains, and beans; soaking nuts and dried fruits; and juicing fruits and vegetables. The mere cooking that is permitted is through a dehydrator. This piece of equipment blasts hot air through the meal but never reaches a temperature greater than 116°F.

Do you have to follow the routine strictly? Of course not. But it is surely worth it to include some of these tactics and ideas in your diet. If you prefer to munch at work, consider carrying in carrots or apple slices. Many of the major grocery shops now provide packaged veggies or fruits that make it easy to pack them and carry them to work. We're a country of convenience, and much of the opposition to better eating is that it does normally take a bit more work and time to purchase and chop fruits and vegetables.

Food merchants have been catching on, slowly, and it is much simpler today to obtain packs of chopped carrots, celery, apples, almonds, and raisins.
Of course, they aren't always organic foods, and organic is the ideal way to go, but we believe anything fresh is immensely superior to cooked, manufactured food.

If you have the time, purchase organic and slice them yourself. But if you're in a rush, and nowhere near a natural food shop, then don't beat yourself up or undermine your efforts since you can't do this 100% all the time. That's not practical. Anything from the fruit and vegetable section is going to be healthier for you than a potato chip, or worse yet, a french fry!

The reason you need a raw food diet?

Because cooking eliminates so many minerals and vitamins from food, you instantly start giving your body what it needs when you stop cooking and start eating raw, nutrient-rich foods. A raw carrot offers tenfold more nourishment than a cooked carrot.

Cooking also affects the chemistry of food, frequently making it more difficult to digest. Why do we have so many stomach issues in our generation?

Because we were putting food into our bodies in a way that we weren't equipped to digest. Fresh items with high fiber and water content relieve constipation from the intestines, cells, and circulatory system. Blockages are cleared and blood flow to every cell in the body is enhanced.

The enhanced blood flow is relevant for two reasons: As discussed above, the blood gives nutrition and oxygen to living cells and transports away their poisonous byproducts.

Obesity is widespread in this generation. The diet business is more lucrative than the oil industry. Why? Because the way we eat and prepare our meals essentially assures that we will overeat. Psychologists tell us that we overeat because our spirit is hungry. But in actuality, our bodies are hungry, even when we feel full. When you start providing your body with the nourishment it needs, you'll quit overeating.

Eating raw food is also a boost for your metabolism. It takes a bit more energy to digest raw food, but it's a healthy procedure. Instead of wasting energy to get rid of pollutants created by heating food, the body utilizes its energy to power every cell, sending forth vitamins, fluids, enzymes, and oxygen to make your body the efficient machine it was made to be.

You will automatically stop overeating since your body and brain will no longer be hungry for the nutrients they require. A hungry brain will stimulate the ideas that induce you to overeat. The brain and the rest of your body don't require quantity; they need quality.

The nourishment of raw food

You may agree on an intellectual level that eating raw foods is a good idea. But does the prospect of leaving a lifetime of eating habits for the sake of what seems like a good idea feel like more than you can do?

So don't! That's dumb and the surest way to ensure you wouldn't even give a raw foods diet a fighting go. Everything is in proportion and we feel that applies to even the healthiest notions. It's not healthy if you can't do it!

Don't conceive of following a raw foods diet as taking anything AWAY. Try adding them in. We think if you put in items like fresh vegetables, sprouts, fruits, and beverages, you won't be as hungry and when you're not hungry, you won't succumb to impulsive eating. If you want that steak or even a

Mcdonald's hamburger, prepare for it and enjoy it. Once you start eating raw foods though and realize how fantastic you feel on them and how much more energy you have, the hamburger just won't look as tasty to you.

You do want to make sure though, that you're consuming enough of the proper forms of nutrients. Eating raw meals doesn't require eating only the raw stuff you love. Watermelon is wonderful for you but is not enough. The same with most meals. You'll need to undertake a little research into which raw foods supply the appropriate proteins, or what combinations of food you need to eat to have enough protein.

Raw food intake is meant to nourish your body in a completely new way, although merely being raw isn't enough. You want to do this to be in balance, and you need to balance the raw foods you're consuming for optimal nutrition.

One approach to guarantee that you are receiving adequate nutrients is to add a different vegetable every week. Buy something you have never heard of, like a leek, or swiss chard. You will discover a whole new world of flavors and sensations open up to you. You will feel more and more discouraged by fast food. I guarantee it.

Does switching to a raw food diet entail never again consuming hot food? Not at all, no. On occasion, you crave something sexy. For many of us, eating a hot meal has always represented comfort. And for the majority of us, carrot sticks or wheatgrass juice won't cut it on a chilly, wet day.

Like our bodies, most raw food is highly perishable. Raw foods begin to rapidly degrade at temperatures exceeding 118 degrees, much as our bodies would if we had a fever that high. Enzymes are food components that can degrade. Our bodies use enzymes to break down food. However, as enzymes are proteins, they have a very distinct three-dimensional spatial structure. This structure may alter if they reach temperatures much higher than 118 degrees.

Enzymes can no longer do the task for which they were intended once they have been subjected to heat. Because cooked foods' enzyme content is compromised and we must produce our enzymes to metabolize them, eating them contributes to chronic sickness.

Cooked food digestion requires important metabolic enzymes, which aid in food digestion. Compared to the digestion of raw food, the digestion of heated food requires a lot more energy. In general, raw food is so much easier to digest than cooked food that it moves through the digestive system in half to a third of the time.

Eating foods devoid of enzymes strains and overworks your pancreas and other organs, eventually wearing them out. After consuming processed foods for their entire lives, many people gradually damage their pancreas and lose the capacity to properly digest their food.

However, if you want your meal to be at least warm, you can certainly steam and blanch things. Cook them to a maximum temperature of 118 degrees Fahrenheit using a food thermometer. The enzymes in food won't be significantly harmed up to this temperature.

Fortunately for those of us newly interested in eating organic and raw foods, there are tons of items out there. Natural and organic foods used to be accessible exclusively at natural food shops, and they might be few and far between. While not as prevalent as Mcdonald's, there ARE many more stand-alone businesses. And supermarket chains are catching on too, with more organic products than ever before. If you don't notice them at your grocery shop, simply ask. You're probably not the only one in your community who wants to see more of these alternatives.

Many grocery shops now display sprouts and other live foods in the produce department. Of course, if they don't, there's nothing simpler to cultivate for yourself than sprouts!

There are also plenty of places on the Web where you may get raw and live foods. Just perform a search on raw foods and you'll come up with several various locations to get the items you'd want to purchase. Many of these sites are also full of good information, to assist you to learn about eating raw foods and to educate you on the individual food qualities.

What else? Experiment with what you like. Take the time to understand a bit about what the various nutrients in foods do for you. A few examples:

Cabbage is High in Vitamin C; necessary for good cell activity
Shiitake mushrooms include vital fatty acids and antioxidants to maintain a healthy immune system
Kale is Rich in fiber and helps decrease calorie intake with reduced hunger. We like that!
Barley – Loaded in niacin, fiber, and iron and is vital for balanced blood sugar.
Pumpkin is So high in fiber and minerals that; helps suppress hunger by filling the stomach with indigestible fibers

Eating Raw food requires drinking less water

When you start eating more raw foods, you may notice you're not as thirsty or don't need as much water or other liquids as you typically do. There are various causes for this.
First of all, raw meals, such as fresh fruits and vegetables, have a larger amount of water in them, so your body is obtaining the hydration it needs from foods.

This doesn't imply you should stop drinking water or drinks. You don't want to accept some of the more extreme components of the raw food craze. First and foremost, listen to your body. It will tell you what it needs. If you're overweight, slow, lethargic, or sad, your body could be asking you to make some dietary adjustments, and raw foods can be one strategy to treat certain physical ailments.

But if you're overweight and have signs of Type II diabetes, extreme thirst might be one indication. When you start eating more raw foods, with a greater fiber and moisture content, you may start to lose weight, and that may go a long way to lowering your blood sugars.

If you're not overweight or don't have Type II diabetes, you still could discover you're not as thirsty as you typically are. First of all, if you're drinking water and juices, you're not drinking coffee, which is extremely dehydrating and makes you thirstier. And by not ingesting as much in the sort of prepared meals or particularly highly processed foods, which have astronomical salt levels, you will be as thirsty either.

By ingesting more raw, uncooked food, and clean water and fruit juices, you're not moving to get your body into equilibrium. Keeping salt to typical amounts found in meals implies you'll start to demand a more balanced quantity of moisture. Don't think of this as altering or taking away. Think of it as providing balance, and it will make the task of eating healthy much simpler.

Why you should avoid processed foods?

Have you ever seen a photograph of your blood plasma after you've eaten a meal from Mcdonald's or Burger King? It's not a nice image. It seems heavy and cloudy. Fast meals are laden with fat and salt. They utilize white bread and buns, which indicates they've used white processed flour, with very little nutrients in them.

And how do you feel after a Big Mac and french fries? Do you need to sleep on TTT? All that fat will pull you down and make you feel lethargic.

Going on a diet is challenging, but think about some of the things you do when you go on a diet. You remove those high-fat, processed, high-sodium items. You eat less, sure.

But you also consume more raw fruits and veggies. You sip water. And the effects of eating in this manner are higher energy, and reduced desire for sleep. Processed meals, with their high-fat content, are hard to digest. They require a significant quantity of the body's energy to consume. When your body's energy isn't spent digesting all that fat, it's available for YOU for work, play, love, and exercise in other words, for LIFE.

These aren't extreme notions. You don't have to make major adjustments to your lifestyle. But take a careful look at what you eat without even thinking about it. We go for the potato chips or stop at Mcdonald's or Taco Bell when we're hungry and we want something fast.

It's a lot simpler these days to keep snacks on hand so you don't have to stop at a fast food business when you're hungry. If you're on the road and feel hungry, pick up a bag of veggies or apple slices at a grocery shop.

Yes, it's quicker to drive up to Wendys, but spending a few additional minutes, not to mention a few extra steps, will be well worth it in energy and vigor.

Raw Food and Skin Health

What's the biggest organ in your body? It's your skin! It offers a protective covering for the various organs of the body. It adjusts to manage your internal body temperature. And is an excellent measure of general health and well-being.

People spend hundreds of dollars on skin preparations to make their skin seem bright and beautiful. They're all topical items that we apply on top of our skin. But if we spent only a portion of the money we spend on these preparations on RAW FOODS, we begin to notice an instant difference in the texture of our skin.

When you consume raw foods, you put more of the critical vitamins and amino acids your body needs into it. You also add moisture organically. Raw foods have a significantly greater moisture content than cooked meals, simply because the cooking process takes off so much important moisture.

Your skin is a reflection of what's going on in the rest of your body. And when your organs and blood are provided the nourishment they require to perform correctly, it appears in your skin. Get your vitamins and hydration from foods like apples and carrots. When you do, then adjectives like inner beauty and inner shine will be ascribed to YOU. Your skin is what's exposed to the rest of the world and healthy, glowing skin gives the finest first impression.

When you start adding raw foods to your diet, things will simply naturally fall into place. You'll feel better. You'll look better. People will respond to you more favorably. You'll have so much more energy for your career, your friends, and your family. And this type of energy is a self-perpetuating phenomenon.

You don't need self-help books and pricey moisturizers and plastic surgery. When your body and skin are receiving their needed nourishment with raw, uncooked foods, you'll look and feel your best, NATURALLY!

Skin tone drinking water, coconut milk, etc.

The greatest method to achieve healthy, beautiful skin is to start from the inside out. Eliminating caffeine in the form of coffee and soda is one approach to start. Caffeine dehydrates the body and skin. And lack of moisture is a proven way to generate lines and wrinkles. It's also a diuretic, generating increased urine flow, again depriving your body and skin of the moisture it requires. We attempt to battle this with moisturizers, but the ideal method is to put the moisture INTO your body, not on it.

Drinking pure water, unprocessed fruit juices, or coconut milk will provide your body and skin the moisture it needs. The colors in fruit juices are the colors of the earth and these colors will reflect themselves in warm and healthy skin tones.

The overall effects of coffee on your body will express themselves in your skin. Heavy caffeine consumers might develop osteoporosis, headaches, melancholy, and insomnia. These may all be reflected in your skin.

When you substitute colas, coffee, and teas produced with boiling water with water, fruit juices, sun tea, and coconut milk, you'll quickly start to feel better and sleep better. Your skin will reflect the wonderful health of all the organs and cells of your body after you've cut the coffee habit.

Another argument for consuming clean water, juices, and sun tea is that when you boil water, you're expelling oxygen from it. When the body rids itself of pollutants, it goes via the skin which is the biggest elimination organ. Raw food enhances your detoxifying rate. Drinking water helps the body clear itself of pollutants. Seaweed is abundant in vitamins and minerals good for the skin and also helps cleanse the body of impurities.

To obtain a healthy complexion, drink lots of water and consume plenty of raw food. What goes into your body is evident in your entire look.

Vegetarian compared to raw food.

What is the difference between vegetarian and raw food diets?

A raw foodist is a vegetarian, but one who normally is not going to cook his veggies or fruits. A vegetarian is someone who just doesn't eat meat, fish, or poultry, but exclusively eats vegetables, pasta, and grains. A vegetarian would eat meatless spaghetti sauce or order onion rings at a restaurant. (Not the healthiest option, but sometimes it's hard to find anything to eat in a restaurant if you're vegetarian much harder if you're a raw foodist.)

There are numerous sorts of vegetarians, such as vegans, or fruitarians, and a raw foodist is a form of vegetarianism. We haven't seen anything about sushi being classified as raw food, although it is. Raw food, nevertheless, typically implies eating raw, uncooked fruits, vegetables, dried fruits, seaweed, etc.

But to be a raw food purist implies raw broccoli, not steamed. To a vegetarian, someone devoted to not consuming meat or fish or animal products, steamed veggies are just as delicious, however, everyone would agree that steaming may take away nutrients from foods, leaving them less nutritious. A vegetarian could ingest dairy or egg products; whereas a vegan will not consume any animal products at all. And a raw foodist is a vegan who eats exclusively uncooked, unadulterated raw foods.

Proponents of the raw diet believe that enzymes are the life energy of a meal and that every food includes its exact blend. These enzymes help us digest meals thoroughly, without depending on our body to manufacture its cocktail of digestive enzymes.

It is also considered that the cooking process damages vitamins and minerals and that cooked meals not only take longer to digest, but also enable partly digested fats, proteins, and carbs to clog up our stomachs and arteries.

Followers of a raw diet assert various health advantages, including:

higher energy levels

enhanced look of skin

better digestion

weight loss

lower risk of heart illness as discussed previously.

Tools for the preparation of raw food

You don't need to make a significant commitment to consuming raw and live foods. You'll probably be saving money by reducing less on overly processed convenience meals. All those high-fat, high-sodium microwaveable meals are pricy, too!

If you're new to this, eating raw foods isn't simply about putting something unusual in your mouth. It's an experience that extends beyond the act of eating. When you're shopping for your meals, make it an aesthetic experience as well. Fill your basket with all the hues of these wonderful living meals.

Invest in an excellent juicer. Numerous catalogs carry these. Shop online. Maybe you might discover a well-used juicer on an auction site. A juicer is NOT a blender. It is significantly more strong since it has to liquefy meals that might be exceedingly fibrous.

You want some decent knives too, for chopping up your fruits and veggies. Invest in a few excellent ones. Turn the labor of slicing up your food into something beautiful.

If you don't have a steamer, invest in one of them also, so you may softly steam your veggies if you wish. Buy particular sorts of steamers. We've seen an asparagus steamer that's expressly intended to steam the woody bottoms more than the sensitive tops.

Get a couple of chopping implements that are also garnishing tools. It is just as simple to chop up carrots using a ridged cutting knife to make them more beautiful. There are specific slicers that make your fruits and vegetables thin and consequently more pleasurable to eat.

And do invest in a new cutting board. You don't want to use the same cutting board for all your fresh new foods that you've used over the years to chop up chicken or other things. No matter how often you scrape, your cutting board may absorb germs. Start anew in all things, not just your meals!

In summary,

If you want a better life, eat more live foods! What are live foods? They are those that have not been altered or changed from their natural state. Also known as raw foods. That is, as produced by the Great Provider.

Living foods are...
Fruits, fresh vegetables, sprouts or sprouts, nuts, and raw seeds without salt, are five extensive families with great variety. If these will predominate in our diets, good health will predominate in our lives. I am not implying that to be healthy and live long days it is necessary to eat only food in its raw state. But I do want to strongly suggest that the less unprocessed food you eat, the better for your health. Some specific recommendations are:

1. Eat more high-water content foods.
2. Properly combine your meals.
3. Eat fruits correctly.

4. Refrain from eating heavy food during certain times of the day (during cycles of assimilation and elimination).
5. Consider your biological adaptation and increase the appropriate amount of live foods in your diet (fruits, vegetables, sprouts, nuts, and seeds).

www.ingramcontent.com/pod-product-compliance
Lightning Source LLC
LaVergne TN
LVHW041300150826
845673LV00008B/2673

* 9 7 9 8 3 6 1 1 4 0 6 2 6 *